10 Steps for Reducing Inflammation

Louis Yandoli

DEDICATION

To my wife, cherished family, my steadfast friends, and all those who have ignited the flame of inspiration along my journey:

This book is a testament to the love, support, and encouragement you all generously offered. Your belief in me has been the bedrock upon which these pages have come to life.

In gratitude and admiration, I dedicate this work to each of you. May it symbolize our shared journey and remind us that we can conquer the highest peaks together. Thank you.

CONTENTS

ABOUT THE AUTHOR

Louis Yandoli is a distinguished professional with over two decades of experience in various consulting and management roles within Global Fortune 500 companies. He holds a bachelor's degree in chemical engineering from Lehigh University and began his career at ExxonMobil, where he was immediately assigned to an international post in Singapore. After a successful four-year stint, particularly in collaborating with clients in Japan, Louis returned to the United States. He pursued a master's degree in engineering, attending classes during evenings and weekends while continuing to work.

In 2013, Louis was awarded a full scholarship to attend Hitotsubashi University in Tokyo, Japan, where he completed his MBA in just one year and graduated at the top of his class. Upon returning to the United States, he transitioned his career to cybersecurity, joining Sony as a Cyber Security Professional.

Louis is passionate about many hobbies, such as cooking, investing, maintaining a healthy lifestyle, acquiring new skills, raising his two young children, and appreciating fine food and wine.

The concept of his "10 Step" series was born out of a conversation with a close friend about sharing knowledge and experiences with others facing similar challenges. Louis hopes that his insights, examples, and wisdom will empower readers to achieve their goals, whatever they may be.

THE 10-STEP APPROACH EXPLAINED

The "10 Steps to Success" book series offers a comprehensive yet easily digestible approach to mastering various skills and topics. Each book in the series follows the same structured format, guiding readers through ten carefully designed steps that build upon one another to create a holistic understanding of the subject matter. This section will explore the standard approach used throughout the "10 Steps to Success" series and explain how this book adheres to the same principles.

1. Embracing the 10-Step Approach

Each "10 Steps to Success" book begins by breaking down a complex subject into ten manageable steps. These steps are designed to be informative and practical, offering readers insights, techniques, and actionable tips they can apply to their lives or work. Focusing on one step at a time allows readers to process and retain the information presented more efficiently, leading to a more effective learning experience.

2. Understanding the Connections Between Steps

While each step in the "10 Steps to Success" series can be valuable on its own, the true power of the approach lies in the connections between the steps. As readers progress through the book, they will find that each step builds upon the previous one, weaving together a cohesive narrative that reinforces key concepts and deepens understanding. By following the steps in sequence, readers can develop a comprehensive and well-rounded mastery of the subject.

3. Efficient and Bite-Sized Learning

The "10 Steps to Success" approach maximizes efficiency by delivering knowledge and information in bite-sized chunks.

Each step is focused and concise, allowing readers to quickly grasp and apply the core concepts in their own lives. This modular format also makes it easy for readers to refer back to specific steps as needed, reinforcing their learning and ensuring they have the tools they need to succeed.

4. Completing the Journey

By working through all ten steps in the "10 Steps to Success" series, readers will thoroughly understand the subject matter and gain the knowledge and skills necessary to succeed in their chosen field or endeavor. In addition, the series provides a clear roadmap for success, guiding readers step by step through the learning process and empowering them to take control of their personal and professional growth.

In summary, the "10 Steps to Success" approach is a proven and effective method for mastering complex subjects and developing new skills. By breaking down topics into manageable steps, connecting the dots between each step, and delivering information in an efficient and digestible format, the series enables readers to deeply understand the subject matter and apply their newfound knowledge to succeed. So, as you embark on your 10-step journey, remember to take your time, trust the process, and enjoy the rewards of mastering a new skill or subject.

5. Personal Experience and Tested Techniques

One of the key strengths of the "10 Steps to Success" series is that the guidance, techniques, and processes presented in each book are not theoretical concepts created in a vacuum. Instead, they are grounded in my personal and professional experiences, accumulated over 20 years of trial and error, learning from mistakes, and refining strategies to optimize outcomes.

Throughout the series, I share my insights and lessons learned from my own experience, offering practical examples and case studies that demonstrate how the 10-step approach has been successfully applied in real-life situations. Then, drawing on these experiences, I hope to provide a relatable and authentic perspective on the subject matter, making it more accessible and engaging for readers.

Moreover, my extensive background in various consulting and management positions across Global Fortune 500 companies has provided a wealth of knowledge and expertise that has been distilled into the "10 Steps to Success" series. This ensures that the advice and techniques offered in each book are relevant, applicable, tested, and proven to deliver results.

As you work through the 10 steps in this book, you can take comfort in knowing that the guidance you are receiving has been honed and refined through years of real-world experience. This practical foundation will help you better understand the concepts and techniques presented and equip you with the confidence and tools necessary to apply them effectively in your professional or personal pursuits.

HELPFUL RESOURCES AND REFERENCES

In this section, I have compiled a selection of books and resources that have greatly influenced and inspired the content of this book. These references, written by experts in the field, provide valuable insights, tips, and techniques that can further enhance your understanding and skills. Each one has helped me immensely in my decades of personal and professional experience thinking through these 10 steps.

Exploring these resources will deepen your knowledge and help you discover additional strategies and ideas to take your knowledge to the next level. Whether you seek more detailed guidance, practical examples, or inspiration from the best in the business, this curated list of resources is an excellent starting point for your continued learning growth.

1. Yates, W. (2020). The Inflammation Nation: The First Clinically Proven Eating Plan to End Our Nation's Secret Epidemic. Free Press.
   - This book presents the first clinically proven eating plan to combat and reverse the inflammatory process that is the basis of many chronic diseases.

2. Sears, B. (2015). The Anti-Inflammation Zone: Reversing the Silent Epidemic That's Destroying Our Health. Harper Collins.
   - Sears discusses how to combat the silent epidemic of inflammation that is gradually damaging our health.

3. Libby, P. (2017). Inflammation in Heart Disease: The Science, The Impact, and The Natural Solutions. Wiley-Blackwell.

- This scientific book provides an overview of the latest research into inflammation's role in heart disease and natural solutions to combat it.

4. Minich, D. M. (2018). Whole Detox: A 21-Day Personalized Program to Break Through Barriers in Every Area of Your Life. HarperOne.
   - This book offers a comprehensive and personalized program to overcome systemic inflammation and balance the body through detox.

5. Ferguson, S. G. (2021). Inflammation Mastery: The Colorful and Definitive Guide for Adults and Kids. Bioactive Publishing.
   - This guide aims to make understanding and managing inflammation simple and accessible for adults and children alike.

6. Jenkins, M., & Jenkins, M. (2020). Your Guide to Understanding Inflammation: Basic Biology, Measurement, Lifestyle and Pharmacological Interventions. Springer.
   - This scientific text provides an in-depth understanding of the biological aspects of inflammation, measurement methods, lifestyle interventions, and pharmacological treatments.

7. Roberts, L. (2021). The Stress-Inflammation Connection: Your Guide to Living an Anti-Inflammatory Lifestyle. Random House.
   - This lifestyle book guides readers on managing stress to reduce inflammation, emphasizing the link between stress and inflammation.

8. Hartung, G. (2017). Anti-Inflammatory Diet: Heal Yourself: The Top 100 Best Recipes For Chronic

Inflammation. Createspace Independent Publishing Platform.

- This book provides the top 100 best recipes tailored to reducing chronic inflammation through dietary change.

9. Pedersen, S. (2012). The Anti-Inflammation Cookbook: The Delicious Way to Reduce Inflammation and Stay Healthy. Chronicle Books.
   - This cookbook promotes a delicious way to reduce inflammation and maintain good health, full of inflammation-fighting recipes.

10. Lipski, E. (2012). Digestive Wellness: Strengthen the Immune System and Prevent Disease Through Healthy Digestion. McGraw-Hill Education.
    - This resource provides an approach to strengthen the immune system and prevent disease through healthy digestion, focusing on reducing inflammation.

11. Laird, L. (2015). The Anti-Inflammatory Kitchen Cookbook: More Than 100 Healing, Low-Histamine, Gluten-Free Recipes. Sterling Epicure.
    - This cookbook shares over 100 healing, gluten-free, and low-histamine recipes to help reduce inflammation.

12. Berndt, C. & Murray, R. (2018). Anti-Inflammatory Diet Slow Cooker Recipes: Prep-and-Go Whole Food Meals. Althea Press.
    - This book combines the convenience of slow cooker meals with a whole food anti-inflammatory diet, providing delicious recipes that reduce inflammation.

13. Chilton, F. H., & Tucker, A. (2018). The Gene Therapy Plan: Taking Control of Your Genetic Destiny with Diet and Lifestyle. Jeremy P. Tarcher/Penguin.
    - This book empowers readers to take control of their genetic destiny through dietary and lifestyle changes to reduce inflammation.

14. Cole, W. (2019). The Inflammation Spectrum: Find Your Food Triggers and Reset Your System. Avery.
    - This book explores the complex relationship between our bodies and the food we eat, outlining a personalized approach to identifying food triggers and rebalancing your system to reduce inflammation.

15. Calimeris, D., & Cook, L. (2017). The Complete Anti-Inflammatory Diet for Beginners: A No-Stress Meal Plan with Easy Recipes to Heal the Immune System. Rockridge Press.
    - This cookbook offers simple, tasty recipes and meal plans designed to help beginners navigate the anti-inflammatory diet and boost their immune system.

16. Babb, M. (2016). Anti-Inflammatory Eating for a Happy, Healthy Brain: 75 Recipes for Alleviating Depression, Anxiety, and Memory Loss. Sasquatch Books.
    - This blend of nutritional guidance and cookbook suggests a diet that alleviates depression, anxiety, and memory loss through anti-inflammatory eating.

17. Calimeris, D., & Bruner, S. (2015). The Anti-Inflammatory Diet & Action Plans: 4-Week Meal Plans to Heal the Immune System and Restore Overall Health. Sonoma Press.

- This comprehensive guide offers four different anti-inflammatory diet plans and recipes to heal the immune system and restore overall health.

18. Goldner, B. (2019). Goodbye Autoimmune Disease: How to Prevent and Reverse Chronic Illness and Inflammatory Symptoms Using Supermarket Foods. Goodbye Lupus.
    - Dr. Goldner shares her expert advice on preventing and reversing chronic illnesses and inflammatory symptoms using foods readily available in supermarkets.

19. Villeponteau, B. (2018). Anti-inflammatory Strategies for Epigenetic Age Reversal. Createspace Independent Publishing Platform.
    - This scientific book delves into anti-inflammatory strategies that aim for age reversal by influencing epigenetic factors.

20. Nordahl, T. (2016). The Nordic Diet: A Beginner's Step-by-Step Guide with Recipes. Skyhorse Publishing.
    - Offers a comprehensive approach to reducing inflammation by adopting a traditional Nordic diet rich in whole foods, fish, berries, and whole grains.

A PERSONAL STORY

As a young and active college student, the last thing you expect to face is a life-changing disease. Yet, it happened to us. I remember it clearly as if it were yesterday. The year was 2005. I was 21, and so was my then-girlfriend Sharon, now my wife. We were in college together, brimming with youthful energy and dreams of our future together. And then, a diagnosis shattered our normality: my wife was diagnosed with rheumatoid arthritis (RA).

If you are familiar with this condition, you understand what a significant impact it can have on a person's life. Rheumatoid arthritis is a chronic inflammatory disorder that affects the joints, causing severe pain, swelling, and stiffness. It was a shock to see my wife, so in love with physical activity, suddenly struggling with everyday things that most of us take for granted. I recall vividly how I had to help her navigate the stairs in her rented home in Lehigh, Pennsylvania, a task that was becoming increasingly challenging for her. Helping her turn on the shower, something she used to do effortlessly, was also becoming a struggle due to her painful joints.

For a while, we felt trapped in this new reality. But gradually, as we delved into understanding her condition and the complex world of inflammation, we found our path to resilience. Our journey became focused on managing her rheumatoid arthritis and reducing the inflammation that was wreaking havoc on her body. We turned to books, the internet, doctors, and eventually to a healthier lifestyle, focusing on diet, physical activity, and an overall reduction in inflammatory activities.

The transformation was not immediate, but the effects were profound. My wife regained control over her body, reducing her RA symptoms significantly. Our combined experience ignited in me a passion for understanding inflammation and how it impacts our lives. And it is this passion that has led me to write this book almost 20 years later.

Inflammation is a double-edged sword. It is an essential part of our body's defensive mechanism, protecting us from injury and infection. However, when inflammation persists longer than necessary, it leads to various health problems - from arthritis and heart diseases to diabetes and cancer. The realization that inflammation was at the root of so many chronic diseases was startling but also empowering. It meant we could potentially manage and even prevent these conditions by controlling inflammation.

Drawing inspiration from the works of notable authors and researchers, I ventured into this complex world, navigating the intersections of science, health, and nutrition. I devoured books like Yates's "The Inflammation Nation," Sears's "The Anti-Inflammation Zone," and Libby's "Inflammation in Heart Disease." They offered profound insights into how the inflammatory process forms the basis of many chronic diseases and how we can combat this silent epidemic.

Cookbooks such as Hartung's "Anti-Inflammatory Diet: Heal Yourself," Pedersen's "The Anti-Inflammation Cookbook," and Laird's "The Anti-Inflammatory Kitchen Cookbook" offered delicious, health-supporting recipes. These books proved instrumental in transforming our kitchen over the years into a hub of anti-inflammatory meals, adding a flavorful spin.

Scientific texts like Jenkins and Jenkins's "Your Guide to Understanding Inflammation" and Villeponteau's "Anti-inflammatory Strategies for Epigenetic Age Reversal" deepened my understanding of the biological aspects of inflammation. They also introduced me to cutting-edge concepts that could help us manage the situation better.

Throughout this journey, we found wisdom, practical tips,

and inspirational stories that transformed our lives and will, hopefully, transform yours too. And that brings me to the primary objective of this book - to share with you these transformative insights, practical strategies, and bite-sized pieces of information to reduce inflammation.

In this book, "10 Steps for Reducing Inflammation," we will explore the vital steps that can lead you toward a healthier, inflammation-free life together. I distill the wealth of knowledge gained from my personal experience and extensive research into this practical guide. This book will help you understand the science behind inflammation, its link with chronic diseases, and its triggers. Most importantly, it will empower you with the tools to control inflammation, focusing on lifestyle changes, diet, stress management, and more.

Through our experience together, we will also delve into delicious recipes that not only tantalize your taste buds but also help you combat inflammation. We will also explore the role of stress in inflammation and how managing it can bring you a step closer to an anti-inflammatory lifestyle.

I hope this book will be your trusted companion in your own path towards an inflammation-free life, just as the referenced authors and researchers have been in mine. Together, we will explore, learn, and progress toward a healthier life. It is time to take the first step towards reducing inflammation. Welcome aboard.

1 UNDERSTANDING INFLAMMATION

What is Inflammation?

Inflammation is a critical part of our body's defense mechanism. Whenever our body experiences harm, whether it is due to an injury, an infection, or exposure to harmful substances, our immune system jumps into action. This response involves mobilizing various cells and chemicals to the site of harm to promote healing and repair.

Acute inflammation, characterized by redness, heat, swelling, pain, and loss of function, is usually short-term and subsides once healing is complete. However, when inflammation becomes chronic or systemic, continuing for extended periods and even without an apparent trigger, it can silently damage tissues over time and contribute to various health problems, including heart disease, diabetes, cancer, and autoimmune disorders like rheumatoid arthritis.

The Biology of Inflammation

The inflammatory process starts with the release of chemicals from damaged tissues. Key stages include:
- The released chemicals cause blood vessels to leak fluid into the tissues, leading to swelling.
- The chemicals attract white blood cells, especially macrophages, to the site of harm.
- The macrophages release further chemicals, including cytokines and growth factors, which stimulate healing but can also prolong the inflammatory response.

Over time, the influx of white blood cells can damage healthy tissues and organs. Moreover, the release of cytokines can trigger a systemic response leading to low-grade, whole-body inflammation. This type of silent inflammation is linked with several chronic diseases, including heart disease, diabetes, and neurodegenerative disorders.

The Impact of Chronic Inflammation

Chronic inflammation poses various potential health risks, making managing and reducing it critical. An integrative approach is emphasized in numerous studies and involves:
- Dietary changes
- Stress management
- Regular physical activity
- Reduction of exposure to environmental toxins

Chronic inflammation can be elusive, often flying under the radar without presenting clear symptoms. However, signs such as persistent fatigue, body pain, skin problems, digestive issues, and high blood pressure can suggest its presence. In addition, inflammatory markers like C-reactive protein (CRP) or cytokines in blood tests can also indicate systemic inflammation.

Inflammation and Lifestyle

Lifestyle plays a crucial role in the prevalence and progression of chronic inflammation. There is a growing body of evidence suggesting that certain habits and lifestyle factors can contribute to sustained inflammation, often without us realizing it. For example, unhealthy dietary habits, a sedentary lifestyle, poor sleep hygiene, chronic stress, and exposure to environmental toxins are all potential triggers of chronic inflammation. Consequently, a comprehensive strategy to combat inflammation needs to address these factors, making necessary adjustments in our daily routines to reduce their inflammatory impact.

Individual Differences in Inflammatory Responses

Our bodies are complex and unique, and how we react to potential inflammatory triggers is no exception. Genetics, age, sex, body composition, and even the composition of our gut microbiota can influence our susceptibility to chronic inflammation and its potential health impacts. Therefore, more than a one-size-fits-all approach is required in managing inflammation. A personalized, individual-centric perspective that considers one's unique biological makeup and lifestyle is integral in effectively addressing inflammation.

Chronic Inflammation and Mental Health

In recent years, a growing body of research has suggested that chronic inflammation may play a significant role in mental health. Furthermore, studies have linked chronic inflammation with several mental health conditions, including depression, anxiety, and cognitive decline. Understanding this connection helps us grasp the widespread impact of chronic inflammation. It reinforces the need for a comprehensive anti-inflammatory approach that addresses physical and mental health.

The Power of an Anti-Inflammatory Diet

Diet plays a pivotal role in modulating inflammation. Certain foods are known to provoke inflammatory responses, while others can help tame it. As we move through this book, we will delve deeper into the concept of an anti-inflammatory diet, understanding the underlying principles, and discovering how we can harness the power of food in our fight against inflammation.

Exercise and Inflammation

Physical activity is another potent tool in our anti-inflammatory arsenal. Regular exercise can help reduce chronic inflammation by promoting a healthy body weight, enhancing immune function, and improving gut health. However, it is not just about the amount of exercise; the type of exercise we engage in can also influence our inflammatory status. This aspect will be discussed in detail in the subsequent steps.

The Role of Stress and Sleep in Inflammation

Chronic stress and poor sleep hygiene can exacerbate inflammation, providing a crucial link between our mental health and physical well-being. Developing effective stress management techniques and cultivating good sleep habits are essential elements of an anti-inflammatory lifestyle, which we will explore further as we proceed.

Setting the Stage for Transformation

In understanding inflammation, we have taken the critical first step toward enhanced health and vitality. The information provided in this step serves as a foundation for building a comprehensive, individualized approach to combat inflammation. As we move forward, we will equip you with the necessary tools and knowledge to identify and address inflammatory triggers in your own life, utilizing the power of diet, physical activity, stress management, and adequate sleep.

In the steps to come, I will provide detailed guidelines on implementing these changes in a sustainable manner, making this approach a practical and enjoyable one. Keep in mind that each small change can make a significant difference, and you are not alone on this path. This journey is a collaborative effort; together, we will navigate the way to an inflammation-free life.

2 RECOGNIZING INFLAMMATION TRIGGERS

One of the most crucial aspects of reducing inflammation lies in understanding its root causes and identifying the triggers that lead to an inflammatory response in your body. While inflammation is a normal, protective response to injury or infection, it becomes a problem when it is chronic or systemic, affecting multiple systems in your body. So, let us explore these triggers and how you can navigate them effectively.

Dietary Triggers: Inflammatory Foods

Certain foods are known to induce inflammation, contributing to various inflammatory diseases. These foods include but are not limited to processed foods, sugary drinks, fried foods, red and processed meats, margarine, shortening, and lard. These foods are often high in trans fats, saturated fats, sugars, and artificial additives, all of which can promote inflammation.

Additionally, foods that you are intolerant or allergic to can cause an inflammatory response. These reactions can vary from person to person, and symptoms can range from mild to severe. Identifying and eliminating these foods from your diet can be a significant step toward reducing inflammation.

Stress: The Silent Inflammatory Trigger

Stress is another significant contributor to inflammation. When you are stressed, your body releases hormones such as cortisol, which prepares your body for a "fight or flight" response. While this is helpful in the short term, chronic stress can lead to an overactive immune system and excessive inflammation.

Understanding your stressors and implementing stress management techniques like mindfulness, yoga, deep breathing, and regular exercise can help regulate your body's stress response and reduce inflammation.

Lack of Sleep: Rest for Recovery

Inadequate sleep can be a potent inflammatory trigger. During sleep, your body performs numerous restorative processes that help regulate inflammation. Lack of sleep can disrupt these processes, leading to increased inflammatory markers.

Ensuring you get sufficient, quality sleep is crucial for managing inflammation. This includes maintaining a regular sleep schedule, optimizing your sleep environment, and addressing any underlying sleep issues such as sleep apnea or insomnia.

Sedentary Lifestyle: Movement Matters

Physical inactivity is often associated with an increased risk of chronic diseases, many of which are linked to inflammation. When we do not move enough, our body's regulatory systems can be thrown off balance, leading to a state of low-grade systemic inflammation. Incorporating regular physical activity into your routine, whether it is walking, jogging, swimming, or resistance training, can help mitigate inflammation.

Environmental Triggers: Toxins and Pollutants

We are constantly exposed to a myriad of environmental toxins and pollutants that can induce inflammation. These include cigarette smoke, air pollution, heavy metals, and chemicals in personal care products and household cleaners, among others. These toxins can induce oxidative stress in our bodies, leading to an inflammatory response.

While it is impossible to completely avoid exposure to these toxins, taking steps to minimize your exposure can be beneficial. This could involve choosing natural personal care and household cleaning products, ensuring good ventilation in your home, and if you smoke, seeking help to quit.

Alcohol and Smoking: Inflammatory Vices

Excessive alcohol consumption and smoking are also inflammatory triggers. Alcohol is metabolically demanding and can lead to inflammation in various tissues, particularly the liver. Similarly, smoking introduces numerous toxins into your body that can cause oxidative stress and inflammation.

Reducing alcohol consumption and eliminating smoking are critical steps in managing inflammation. If you need help with these changes, do not hesitate to seek professional assistance. There are numerous resources and support networks available to help you navigate these challenges.

Medication-Induced Inflammation: Side Effects and Sensitivities

Certain medications can induce inflammation as a side effect or due to an allergic reaction. If you suspect a medication you are taking is contributing to your inflammation, it's important not to discontinue it abruptly. Instead, discuss your concerns with your healthcare provider. They can help determine if the medication is the culprit and discuss potential alternatives or strategies to manage this side effect.

Gut Health: The Microbiome-Inflammation Connection

Finally, an often overlooked but significant source of inflammation is your gut health. Your gut is home to trillions of bacteria, fungi, viruses, and other microbes collectively known as the microbiome. A healthy microbiome is crucial for maintaining an optimal immune response and keeping inflammation in check.

However, an imbalance in the gut microbiome, often termed as 'dysbiosis,' can contribute to chronic inflammation. This imbalance can be triggered by a poor diet, stress, lack of sleep, certain medications, and other factors. By addressing these triggers and promoting a healthy microbiome through diet, probiotics, and other lifestyle interventions, you can significantly impact your body's inflammatory response.

Recognizing and understanding these triggers can be a powerful tool in your journey toward reducing inflammation. In the next step, we will delve into dietary strategies to combat inflammation, where you will learn about the types of foods that can either increase or decrease inflammation and how to make informed choices that promote your health and well-being.

3 AN ANTI-INFLAMMATORY DIET

The Core of Anti-Inflammatory Living: Dietary Choices

The food we consume plays a pivotal role in our health. Our dietary choices can either initiate a cascading cycle of inflammation or quell it, thereby directly influencing our state of health and wellness. This makes diet the cornerstone of an anti-inflammatory lifestyle.

Modern research has shed light on how our daily intake of food affects our bodily functions, specifically the immune responses. Chronic inflammation is now identified as a significant contributing factor to many non-communicable diseases, such as heart disease, diabetes, and arthritis. On a molecular level, certain foods can provoke an inflammatory response, while others can dampen it.

Inflammation is not a solitary health issue; it is deeply connected to our overall well-being. It is also increasingly being linked to mental health conditions, including depression and cognitive decline. This tells us that our food choices can influence not just our physical health but our mental and emotional wellness as well.

Transitioning to an anti-inflammatory diet can be a powerful strategy to combat chronic inflammation, thus promoting overall health and preventing a host of diseases. It is an invitation to explore diverse foods, experiment with new recipes, and enjoy meals that nourish our bodies and soothe our minds.

The Foundations of an Anti-Inflammatory Diet

At its core, an anti-inflammatory diet revolves around foods that prevent or reduce inflammation. These are foods that are nutrient-dense and packed with elements that our bodies need to function optimally. Conversely, it means avoiding foods that promote inflammation.

Pro-inflammatory foods typically include processed foods loaded with sugars, unhealthy fats, and artificial additives. These foods are low in nutrients and high in components that can trigger inflammation. Regular consumption of such foods can lead to a state of chronic inflammation, which is detrimental to our health.

In contrast, anti-inflammatory foods are rich in nutrients that can tame inflammation. They include colorful fruits and vegetables, lean proteins, whole grains, healthy fats, and various other foods that naturally control inflammation. Such a diet is dense in antioxidants, fiber, and anti-inflammatory fats, helping us to maintain a healthy immune system and prevent disease.

Embracing an anti-inflammatory diet does not require an abrupt overhaul of eating habits. Instead, it is a gradual process that involves small, consistent changes. The goal is not to achieve perfection but to progressively shift towards eating patterns that support health and mitigate inflammation.

The Rainbow Diet: An Array of Fruits and Vegetables

A vital element of an anti-inflammatory diet is a variety of fruits and vegetables. The broader the spectrum of colors you consume, the wider the range of nutrients you get. These plant foods are loaded with powerful antioxidants and anti-inflammatory compounds that help neutralize free radicals and curb inflammation.

Every fruit and vegetable color signifies the presence of different nutrients, each offering unique health benefits. For instance, green leafy vegetables like spinach and kale are rich in vitamin K and fiber, which are known to mitigate inflammation. Similarly, brightly colored fruits like berries are packed with anthocyanins, a type of antioxidant with potent anti-inflammatory effects.

Aim to incorporate a mix of different fruits and vegetables into your daily meals. Experiment with seasonal produce and try new varieties. The goal is to paint your plate with as many colors as possible, turning each meal into a feast of nutrients that supports your body's anti-inflammatory defenses.

Whole Grains and Fiber-Rich Foods: The Unsung Heroes

Whole grains and fiber-rich foods form another critical part of an anti-inflammatory diet. Foods like brown rice, quinoa, oats, and whole-grain bread are excellent sources of dietary fiber, which has been linked to a reduced risk of inflammation-associated conditions like cardiovascular disease and type 2 diabetes.

Dietary fiber aids digestion, helps maintain a healthy weight, and keeps blood sugar levels stable - all of which contribute to controlling inflammation. Moreover, fiber also supports a healthy gut microbiome, which plays an essential role in immune function and inflammation regulation.

Switching from refined grains to whole grains is a simple yet powerful step toward anti-inflammatory eating. So next time you are shopping for bread, pasta, or rice, consider opting for the whole-grain version.

Lean Proteins and Healthy Fats: Balancing the Nutrient Puzzle

While plant foods are the primary focus of an anti-inflammatory diet, lean proteins and healthy fats also play a crucial role. Proteins are essential for cell repair, immune function, and muscle health, while healthy fats, especially omega-3 fatty acids, are renowned for their anti-inflammatory properties.

Fish like salmon, mackerel, and sardines, along with flaxseeds and walnuts, are excellent sources of omega-3s. On the other hand, lean proteins can come from both animal sources like poultry, fish, and low-fat dairy and plant sources such as lentils, chickpeas, and quinoa.

Spice Up Your Diet: The Power of Herbs and Spices

Beyond merely adding flavor to your meals, herbs and spices are nutritional powerhouses that boast significant anti-inflammatory properties. Curcumin in turmeric, for instance, has been extensively studied for its potent anti-inflammatory effects. Similarly, ginger contains compounds like gingerols and shogaols, which are known to suppress inflammation and offer analgesic effects.

Other spices like cinnamon, garlic, cayenne, and black pepper have been shown to reduce inflammation and support overall health. Herbs such as rosemary, thyme, and oregano are not just flavor enhancers but also carry an array of antioxidants that help combat oxidative stress and inflammation.

Incorporating these herbs and spices into your cooking not only elevates your culinary experiences but also significantly boosts the anti-inflammatory potential of your meals. Experiment with these aromatic treasures in your recipes and discover new flavors while reaping their health benefits.

Hydration: An Essential Aspect of Anti-Inflammatory Living

Water is often overlooked in nutrition discussions, but it is an essential component of an anti-inflammatory lifestyle. Adequate hydration helps maintain the function of every system in your body, including your heart, brain, and muscles. It aids digestion, carries nutrients to your cells, provides a moist environment for ear, nose, and throat tissues, and flushes toxins from your body.

While the amount of water required may vary based on various factors like age, gender, activity level, and climate, a good rule of thumb is to drink at least eight 8-ounce glasses of water per day. You can also obtain hydration from fruits and vegetables rich in water, herbal teas, and broths.

Beyond Diet: Lifestyle Factors Complementing Anti-Inflammatory Eating

While diet is the cornerstone of an anti-inflammatory lifestyle, it does not work in isolation. Lifestyle factors such as exercise, sleep, stress management, and avoidance of harmful substances like tobacco and excessive alcohol also play a vital role in regulating inflammation.

Regular physical activity has been shown to lower inflammation, improve immune function, and reduce the risk of chronic diseases. Adequate sleep allows the body to rest, repair, and recover, supporting the immune system and reducing inflammation. Stress management techniques like mindfulness, meditation, and yoga can help decrease the production of stress hormones, which in turn helps lower inflammation.

An anti-inflammatory lifestyle, therefore, is an integrative approach that combines a nutrient-dense diet with a balanced lifestyle.

In the next section, we will discuss the importance of personalized nutrition in implementing an anti-inflammatory diet and how small, gradual changes can lead to significant health transformations over time.

Personalized Nutrition: There is no one-size-fits-all diet

When it comes to anti-inflammatory eating, it is crucial to remember that everyone's body responds differently to various foods. While the foods discussed so far generally have anti-inflammatory properties, the optimal diet may vary for each individual. Some people might have food sensitivities or allergies that can actually trigger inflammation - even to foods considered "healthy" or "anti-inflammatory."

For this reason, a personalized approach to nutrition is often the best strategy. Listen to your body, understand how it responds to different foods, and adjust your diet accordingly. Professional guidance from a registered dietitian or a healthcare provider could also provide valuable insights and help tailor your diet to your specific needs and preferences.

The Power of Incremental Change: Start Small, Transform Big

Adopting an anti-inflammatory lifestyle does not necessitate sweeping, radical changes to your existing habits. Instead, it can be approached through small, manageable shifts in your diet and lifestyle that can gradually accumulate into profound health transformations.

Start with simple steps such as adding one extra serving of fruits or vegetables to your meals, switching from refined to whole grains, or incorporating a brief walk or exercise routine into your day. Over time, these small changes can add up, eventually steering you towards a comprehensive anti-inflammatory lifestyle.

A Journey Towards Holistic Health

An anti-inflammatory lifestyle is less about stringent rules and more about understanding the profound impact of your diet and lifestyle choices on your health. By embracing a diet rich in anti-inflammatory foods and maintaining a balanced lifestyle, you can harness the power of nutrition to control inflammation and foster overall well-being.

As we delve deeper into subsequent steps in this book, we will unravel more detailed strategies and tips to further support your journey. However, always remember - the goal is not perfection but progress. Every small step you take towards an anti-inflammatory lifestyle is a victory worth celebrating.

In our next step, we will delve into the world of gut health - an often underappreciated aspect of controlling inflammation. We will explore the importance of a healthy gut microbiome, the influence of probiotics and prebiotics, and the role of gut health in inflammation and immune function. Stay tuned.

4 MEAL PLANNING

The Importance of Meal Planning

When it comes to reducing inflammation through diet, meal planning is an essential tool. It can ensure that you consistently make healthier food choices, keep track of what you eat, and prevent impulsive eating habits that might derail your anti-inflammatory goals. By dedicating a little bit of time each week to plan out your meals, you are making an investment in your health. Not only can meal planning help you incorporate anti-inflammatory foods into your diet, but it can also help to reduce food waste, save time on grocery shopping, and minimize the stress of figuring out what to eat each day.

Understanding the Anti-Inflammatory Food Pyramid

The anti-inflammatory food pyramid is a helpful guide when planning your meals. This pyramid prioritizes foods known to have anti-inflammatory effects while minimizing those that can promote inflammation.

At the base of the pyramid are fruits and vegetables, which should form the bulk of your meals. These foods are high in antioxidants and fiber, which help reduce inflammation. Next, you will find whole grains, lean proteins (such as fish and chicken), and plant-based protein sources like beans and lentils. Further up the pyramid, there are healthy fats, like those found in avocados, nuts, seeds, and olive oil. These foods contain monounsaturated fats and omega-3 fatty acids, both of which have been shown to have anti-inflammatory properties. At the top of the pyramid are foods that should be consumed sparingly, such as red meat, processed foods, and sugar-sweetened beverages.

Choosing the Right Ingredients

Knowing what to look for when shopping for anti-inflammatory ingredients is critical. Whole foods should be your primary focus, as they are rich in the nutrients your body needs to fight inflammation. These include fruits, vegetables, whole grains, lean proteins, and healthy fats. Consider incorporating the following nutrient-rich, anti-inflammatory foods into your meals:

- Berries: Berries like strawberries, blueberries, and raspberries are rich in antioxidants, particularly anthocyanins, which have been shown to reduce inflammation.
- Fatty fish: Salmon, sardines, mackerel, and other fatty fish are high in omega-3 fatty acids, potent anti-inflammatory nutrients.
- Leafy green vegetables: Foods like spinach, kale, and collard greens are high in antioxidants and other anti-inflammatory compounds.
- Olive oil: Extra virgin olive oil contains monounsaturated fats and a compound called oleocanthal, which has been likened to the anti-inflammatory action of ibuprofen.
- Nuts and seeds: These are excellent sources of healthy fats, fiber, and antioxidants.

By focusing on these ingredients and avoiding processed foods, sugars, and unhealthy fats, you are setting the stage for a diet that supports a reduced inflammation level.

Creating Balanced, Nutrient-Dense Meals

The next step in meal planning is creating balanced meals. Each meal should include a good mix of proteins, carbohydrates, and fats to provide a steady release of energy throughout the day and keep you satiated. A balanced meal also ensures you are getting a wide array of nutrients needed to support overall health and combat inflammation.

A helpful tool for creating balanced meals is the plate method. Imagine your plate divided into quarters. Fill half your plate with colorful vegetables, one quarter with lean or plant-based proteins, and the final quarter with whole grains or other complex carbohydrates. Add a small amount of healthy fat, like a drizzle of olive oil over your veggies, some avocado slices, or a handful of nuts or seeds.

Exploring Anti-Inflammatory Recipes

The beauty of an anti-inflammatory diet is that it does not mean you have to sacrifice flavor. There are countless delicious, nutrient-dense recipes available that align with an anti-inflammatory eating plan. Look for recipes that feature the foods we have discussed, and feel free to experiment with new ingredients or cooking methods.

When planning your meals for the week, try to include a variety of foods to ensure you are getting a broad spectrum of nutrients. This also helps prevent mealtime boredom, making you more likely to stick to your healthy eating plan.

A sample day's menu might look like this:
- Breakfast: Overnight oats topped with a mix of berries and a sprinkle of chia seeds.
- Lunch: Grilled salmon salad with mixed greens, cherry tomatoes, cucumber, avocado, and an olive oil-lemon vinaigrette.
- Snack: A handful of almonds and a piece of fresh fruit.
- Dinner: Quinoa-stuffed bell peppers with a side of steamed broccoli.

Meal Prep: Your Time-Saving Strategy

Meal prep is a technique that involves preparing meals or meal components ahead of time. It is a great way to save time during the week and make it easier to stick to your anti-inflammatory diet. You might choose to prep all of your meals for the week or prepare some ingredients (like chopping veggies, cooking grains, or roasting proteins) to make cooking meals faster and easier throughout the week. Having ready-to-eat meals or prepped ingredients in your fridge reduces the temptation to opt for quick, processed food options, which often contribute to inflammation.

Now let us discuss other important considerations such as portion control and the role of hydration in an anti-inflammatory diet. Furthermore, we will delve into the importance of mindful eating and its connection to inflammation. Remember, it is not just about changing what you eat; it is about changing your relationship with food.

Mindful Eating: Enjoyment and Satisfaction

Mindful eating is an approach that involves paying full attention to your food as you eat it, noting the flavors, textures, and smells, and listening to your body's hunger and fullness cues. It is a simple yet powerful practice that can help you make healthier choices and enjoy the foods you eat even more.

In the context of an anti-inflammatory diet, mindful eating can be particularly beneficial. It can help you tune into your body and notice how different foods affect you. For instance, you may realize that certain foods make you feel more energetic, while others might seem to trigger symptoms of inflammation. Over time, these insights can guide you in shaping your diet to support your health better.

Moreover, mindful eating can promote healthier eating behaviors, such as slower eating and more thoughtful food choices, which can further contribute to reducing inflammation.

Understanding Portion Sizes

While focusing on nutrient-dense, anti-inflammatory foods is essential; it is also crucial to be mindful of portion sizes.

Even healthy foods can contribute to unwanted weight gain and potentially increased inflammation if eaten in excess.

A practical way to manage portion sizes is by using your hand as a guide:

- Your fist is about the same size as one serving of vegetables or fruit.
- Your palm represents a good serving size for protein.
- Your cupped hand equates to a serving of cooked grains or starchy vegetables.
- Your thumb is about the size of a serving of fat, like oils, nuts, or seeds.

Remember, these are general guidelines, and individual needs can vary based on factors like age, sex, weight, and activity level.

The Role of Hydration

Water plays a fundamental role in nearly all bodily functions, including digestion and nutrient absorption, both crucial in managing inflammation. Adequate hydration helps flush toxins out of the body, supports the health of your cells, and even aids in the transportation of anti-inflammatory compounds to where they are needed in the body.

Aim for at least eight 8-ounce glasses of water a day, but remember that needs can vary widely depending on factors like climate, physical activity, and individual metabolism. Foods, especially fruits and vegetables, also contribute to your hydration status.

Anti-Inflammatory Spices and Herbs

Remember the power of spices and herbs. Many have potent anti-inflammatory properties and can be easily incorporated into your meals. Turmeric, for instance, contains curcumin, a compound with potent anti-inflammatory effects. Ginger, cinnamon, garlic, and rosemary also offer similar benefits.

Not only do they enhance the flavor of your meals, but they also boost your dishes' anti-inflammatory potential.

Cooking Techniques Matter

Another crucial aspect of preparing anti-inflammatory meals is the cooking methods used. Different techniques can influence the nutrient content of your food and its overall effect on inflammation. For instance, overcooking vegetables can lead to significant nutrient loss, diminishing their anti-inflammatory properties.

Grilling, roasting, and frying at high temperatures can lead to the formation of advanced glycation end products (AGEs), which have been linked to increased inflammation and chronic disease. In contrast, methods like steaming, boiling, or baking at lower temperatures tend to produce fewer AGEs. Also, slow cookers are an excellent tool for cooking at low temperatures over more extended periods.

Incorporating raw fruits and vegetables into your diet is another way to maximize nutrient intake. Salads, smoothies, and fresh salsas are delicious ways to enjoy raw produce.

Balancing Macros in Your Meals

While this book primarily emphasizes the types of foods you should include in your diet for their anti-inflammatory properties, it is essential to remember that the balance of macronutrients - carbohydrates, protein, and fat - also matters.

Try to include a source of protein, healthy fats, and complex carbohydrates in each meal. Protein is necessary for repairing body tissues, fats provide a concentrated source of energy and help you absorb fat-soluble vitamins, and carbohydrates are your body's primary energy source.

While carbohydrates are essential, it is important to choose mostly complex carbohydrates like whole grains, legumes, and starchy vegetables, which are digested slowly and have less of an impact on blood sugar levels. Refined carbohydrates like white bread, pasta, and sugary foods can cause rapid spikes in blood sugar and contribute to inflammation.

Shopping Smart

Planning and preparing anti-inflammatory meals start with intelligent shopping. Here are a few tips to help you navigate the grocery store:

- Shop the perimeter: The perimeter of the grocery store is where fresh foods like fruits, vegetables, dairy, meat, and fish are usually located. Most of your shopping should be focused here.
- Read labels: Avoid foods with a long list of ingredients, especially if you cannot pronounce them or do not know what they are. These are often processed foods that are high in sugar and unhealthy fats.
- Choose whole grains: Look for words like "whole grain" or "100% whole wheat" on bread and pasta labels. If the word "whole" is missing, it is likely made from refined grains.
- Buy in season: Fruits and vegetables are often cheaper and fresher when bought in season.

Shopping smart is the first step to eating an anti-inflammatory diet. By filling your cart with nutrient-dense foods, you will be well on your way to preparing delicious, health-promoting meals.

Closing Thoughts:

Planning and preparing anti-inflammatory meals can feel like a daunting task, but it is well worth the effort. By eating a diet rich in whole, nutrient-dense foods, practicing mindful eating, and understanding portion sizes, you can significantly reduce inflammation in your body. Incorporating anti-inflammatory herbs and spices, choosing beneficial cooking methods, and balancing macronutrients are additional steps that contribute to a holistic, well-rounded approach to an anti-inflammatory diet. The upcoming steps will continue to guide you on this journey toward a healthier, inflammation-free lifestyle.

5 INTEGRATING PHYSICAL ACTIVITY

The Role of Exercise in Reducing Inflammation

Exercise plays a critical role in managing inflammation in the body. While it may seem counterintuitive, given that intense physical activity can cause temporary inflammation, the long-term effects of a regular exercise routine are decidedly anti-inflammatory. When you exercise, your body produces certain proteins known as cytokines, which have anti-inflammatory properties. Exercise also helps to reduce levels of inflammation-inducing chemicals, such as TNF alpha and IL-6. Moreover, physical activity assists in weight management, which is crucial because obesity is a known factor contributing to systemic inflammation.

Different Types of Exercise

Physical activities can be broadly divided into three categories: aerobic exercises, strength training, and flexibility exercises. Each type offers unique benefits and can help reduce inflammation in various ways.

1. Aerobic Exercises: Also known as cardio, these exercises increase your heart rate and breathing. Regular aerobic exercise reduces inflammation by improving circulation and helping your immune system function more effectively. Examples include brisk walking, running, swimming, cycling, and dancing.
2. Strength Training: These exercises help build muscle mass. Having more muscle mass helps control body fat, reducing inflammation caused by obesity. Strength training exercises include lifting weights, using resistance bands, or doing bodyweight exercises like squats and push-ups.
3. Flexibility Exercises: These exercises help maintain joint health and prevent injuries, reducing

inflammation caused by joint disorders like arthritis. Yoga and stretching routines are typical examples of flexibility exercises.

Each of these types of exercise contributes to your overall health in different ways, so a balanced exercise routine should include a mix of all three.

The Importance of Consistency and Moderation

Starting an exercise routine is often the most challenging part. It is important to remember that consistency is more important than intensity when you are starting. It is better to exercise regularly, even if you can only manage light or moderate activity, rather than exercising intensely but inconsistently.

On the other hand, it is also essential to do it sparingly. Excessive, intense exercise can lead to injuries and, ironically, increased inflammation. Listening to your body and giving it time to rest and recover is just as important as the exercise itself.

Incorporating Exercise into Your Daily Routine

Finding ways to incorporate physical activity into your everyday life is a great way to ensure consistency. It can be as simple as choosing the stairs over the elevator, biking or walking to work instead of driving or doing light exercises during your lunch break. Remember, every bit of physical activity counts.

Creating an Exercise Routine

Designing an exercise routine can seem daunting, but it does not have to be. A few considerations can help you create a routine that suits your lifestyle, fitness level, and preferences:

- Frequency: Aim to exercise most days of the week. According to the CDC, adults should aim for at least 150 minutes of moderate-intensity or 75 minutes of high-intensity aerobic activity per week, along with muscle-strengthening activities on two or more days a week.
- Type: As mentioned earlier, a balanced exercise routine includes a mix of aerobic exercises, strength training, and flexibility exercises. You can choose activities you enjoy to make your routine more fun and sustainable.
- Time: Decide on a convenient time to exercise and try to stick to it. You are more likely to stay consistent if you incorporate exercise into your daily schedule.
- Progression: Start slow and gradually increase the intensity of your workouts as your fitness level improves. This approach will help prevent injuries and make your routine more manageable.

Starting an exercise routine is a significant step in reducing inflammation and improving your overall health. Remember, it is always advisable to consult with a healthcare professional or a fitness expert before starting a new exercise routine, especially if you have a chronic health condition or have not been physically active for a long time. They can help you understand your limits and guide you to make safe and beneficial exercise choices.

The Connection between Mental Health and Exercise

Physical activity does not just affect your physical health - it also has profound impacts on your mental well-being. Regular exercise is known to reduce stress, anxiety, and depression, all of which can contribute to systemic inflammation. The "feel-good" hormones released during and after exercise can help improve your mood and sleep quality, further assisting in controlling inflammation.

Exercises like yoga and tai chi also incorporate mindfulness and deep breathing, which can reduce mental stress and thereby decrease inflammation. If you enjoy the mind-body connection these types of exercise offer, consider making them a regular part of your routine.

Overcoming Barriers to Exercise

As beneficial as physical activity can be for your health, there can be barriers that prevent you from exercising regularly. These could range from lack of time and motivation to physical limitations or lack of access to facilities. It is essential to identify these barriers and find practical ways to overcome them.

For those with time constraints, consider incorporating exercise into your daily routine. For instance, take the stairs instead of the elevator, park your car farther from the door, or take a brisk walk during your lunch break. Remember, even small amounts of exercise can add up over the day.

If motivation is an issue, finding an exercise buddy can make workouts more enjoyable and help you stick to your routine. For those with physical limitations, low-impact exercises such as water aerobics or chair exercises can be excellent alternatives. And if access to a gym or equipment is a problem, there are numerous practical exercises that require no equipment and can be done at home.

Importance of Rest and Recovery

Just as consistent physical activity is crucial to managing inflammation, so is allowing your body time to rest and recover. Rest days are essential to prevent overuse injuries, give your muscles time to repair and strengthen, and keep you from feeling burned out. Over-exercising without adequate rest can actually contribute to inflammation rather than alleviate it.

Listen to your body's signals. If you are feeling fatigued or experiencing prolonged muscle soreness, it may be your body's way of telling you to slow down. Incorporating relaxation techniques such as yoga and mindfulness-based stress reduction can also aid in recovery and help manage inflammation.

Building a Lifelong Habit

Remember, the goal is not just to exercise for a few weeks or months — it is to make physical activity a permanent part of your lifestyle. Start small, set realistic goals, and gradually increase your activity level. Celebrate your successes, no matter how small they may seem. The benefits of physical activity are cumulative and develop over time.

Just as you have learned to incorporate anti-inflammatory foods into your diet, learning to integrate regular physical activity into your life is a skill. With practice and patience, you can make it a habit — one that has the power to significantly reduce inflammation and enhance your overall quality of life.

We have now completed our discussion on the role of physical activity in reducing inflammation. In the next step, we will explore another vital aspect of your anti-inflammation journey: the importance of managing stress.

6 MANAGING STRESS

Understanding the Link between Stress and Inflammation

In our journey through understanding and combating inflammation, we have discussed the importance of diet, identifying triggers, and physical activity. Now, we turn our attention to an often-overlooked yet significant component - stress.

Stress is not just an emotional or psychological state. It is a physiological response that can trigger inflammation in the body. When we experience stress, our bodies produce chemicals like cortisol and adrenaline, which can drive up inflammation levels. Therefore, effectively managing stress can be a powerful tool in our anti-inflammatory toolbox.

Identifying Sources of Stress

The first step towards managing stress is to identify the sources of stress in your life. This can be anything from a high-pressure job, a tumultuous relationship, financial worries, or even daily hassles like a long commute. It is important to note that stress is not solely derived from negative circumstances; even positive events like a wedding or a job promotion can induce stress. Once you identify your stressors, you can take strategic steps to manage them.

Incorporating Relaxation Techniques

Relaxation techniques can help calm your mind, reduce stress hormones, and lower your heart rate. Many of these techniques have also been shown to have anti-inflammatory effects. There are many relaxation methods to explore, and different approaches work for different people. It is important to find a method that fits you and your lifestyle. Here are a few techniques you may consider:

- **Meditation:** Numerous studies have shown that regular meditation can reduce inflammation. Mindfulness meditation has been shown to lower levels of inflammatory markers. As a practice, meditation involves focusing your attention and eliminating the stream of jumbled thoughts that may be crowding your mind and causing stress.
- **Deep Breathing:** Deep breathing, or diaphragmatic breathing, involves fully engaging the diaphragm, a muscle located horizontally between the thoracic cavity and the abdominal cavity. Deep breathing has been found to reduce stress and create a sense of calm and can be done anywhere, anytime.
- **Progressive Muscle Relaxation:** This technique involves slowly tensing and then releasing each muscle group in the body. By focusing on the difference between muscle tension and relaxation, you can become more aware of physical sensations, promoting overall relaxation and stress reduction.
- **Yoga and Tai Chi:** These forms of gentle exercise incorporate breath control, meditation, and specific movements or postures. Both have been found to reduce stress and inflammation.

Each of these techniques can be incorporated into your daily routine. It may take time to learn these techniques and achieve noticeable results, so be patient with yourself. Over time, you will become more adept at using these techniques and they can become an integral part of your stress management toolkit.

Enhancing Sleep Quality

Sleep and stress have an interconnected relationship. Chronic stress can lead to sleep disturbances, while inadequate or poor-quality sleep can exacerbate stress levels. Additionally, chronic sleep deprivation is linked to higher levels of systemic inflammation. By prioritizing sleep and implementing good sleep hygiene, you can improve both your stress levels and inflammation.

Establish a regular sleep schedule by going to bed and waking up at the same time each day. Make your sleeping environment as comfortable as possible by keeping it cool, dark, and quiet. Also, try to avoid stimulating activities and electronics before bedtime as they can interfere with your body's natural sleep-wake cycle.

Physical Activity for Stress Management

We have previously covered the importance of physical activity for reducing inflammation, but it is worth noting its role in stress management. Regular exercise can lower stress hormones, boost mood, improve sleep quality, and act as a natural anti-inflammatory. The key is to find an activity you enjoy and make it a part of your daily routine.

Cognitive Behavioral Strategies

Cognitive-behavioral strategies can be particularly effective for stress management. These techniques involve changing the way you think about stress and developing healthier responses to stressful situations. Cognitive restructuring, for example, helps you to identify and challenge stress-inducing thought patterns and replace them with more balanced views.

Another sound cognitive-behavioral strategy is problem-solving. If certain situations or issues are causing you stress, work on developing a plan to address them. Breaking down the problem into smaller, manageable parts can make it seem less overwhelming and give you a sense of control over the situation.

Nurturing Social Connections

Humans are social creatures, and strong, supportive relationships can be a powerful buffer against stress. Social connections can provide emotional support, improve feelings of self-worth, and create a sense of belonging, all of which can help you manage stress. Be available for the people who are important to you. This could be sharing a meal, having a chat, or participating in shared activities.

The Role of Professional Support

While self-care strategies for stress management can be highly effective, it is also crucial to recognize when professional help might be necessary. If stress is overwhelming and interfering with your daily life, or if you are struggling with mental health issues such as depression or anxiety, do not hesitate to seek professional help. Mental health professionals can provide additional tools and strategies for managing stress and improving your well-being.

Remember, reducing stress is not just about feeling better in the moment. It is about enhancing your overall health and taking a proactive stance against chronic inflammation. As with every step in our anti-inflammatory trip, patience and consistency are crucial. Implementing these techniques is a process, but with time, they can become habitual and significantly enhance your quality of life.

In the next step, we will move on to discuss another important aspect of an anti-inflammatory lifestyle - understanding and managing environmental factors that can contribute to inflammation. Stay with us on this journey as we continue to explore holistic ways to combat inflammation and improve our well-being.

7 THE ENVIRONMENT AND INFLAMMATION

The Connection Between Environment and Inflammation

It is important to understand that our environment plays a significant role in our overall health. In addition to diet, exercise, and stress, exposure to certain environmental factors can contribute to chronic inflammation. The air we breathe, the water we drink, and the products we use daily can all contain toxins and pollutants that exacerbate inflammation in our bodies. These toxins, also known as environmental endocrine disruptors (EEDs), can interfere with our endocrine system, contributing to an array of health issues, including inflammation.

Air Quality and Inflammation

Air pollution is a significant contributor to systemic inflammation. When we inhale pollutants, such as particulate matter, nitrogen oxides, and volatile organic compounds, they can interact with the cells in our respiratory tract and trigger an inflammatory response. Over time, this can lead to chronic inflammation and associated diseases like asthma, allergies, and cardiovascular disease.

Improving the air quality in your surroundings is a critical step in reducing inflammation. This can involve ensuring proper ventilation in your home, using air purifiers, and limiting time spent in heavily polluted areas. Regular cleaning can also help reduce indoor pollutants such as dust mites and mold, which can trigger inflammatory responses, especially in people with allergies.

Water Quality and Inflammation

Just like the air we breathe, the water we consume can be a source of toxins and pollutants. Water contaminated with heavy metals, pesticides, or microplastics can increase our body's toxic load and contribute to inflammation. Ensuring that your drinking water is clean and safe is, therefore, crucial.

To improve your water quality, consider investing in a high-quality water filter that can remove potential contaminants. Also, be mindful of the containers you use to store your water. Opt for glass or stainless steel over plastic, which can leach harmful chemicals into your water.

Reducing Exposure to Toxins in Personal Care and Household Products

Many of the personal care and household products we use daily, from cosmetics to cleaning supplies, can contain harmful chemicals that contribute to inflammation. These can include parabens, phthalates, and synthetic fragrances, which have been linked to hormone disruption and inflammation.

Reducing your exposure to these toxins involves making mindful choices about the products you use. Opt for products with natural ingredients and avoid those containing harmful chemicals. Reading labels can help you make informed decisions.

In the next part of this step, we will discuss more ways to reduce your exposure to environmental toxins, including dietary modifications and lifestyle changes. Remember, every small step towards a cleaner and safer environment can make a significant difference in reducing inflammation and improving your overall health.

Dietary Exposure to Environmental Toxins

Our daily diet is another potential source of exposure to environmental toxins. These toxins can come from various sources, such as pesticides and herbicides used in farming, hormones, and antibiotics used in animal husbandry, and the packaging used for food products. Persistent organic pollutants (POPs), such as polychlorinated biphenyls (PCBs) and dioxins, are also known to bioaccumulate in the food chain and can trigger inflammatory responses.

You can significantly reduce dietary exposure to these toxins by adopting a few mindful eating practices. Primarily, aim to consume organic fruits and vegetables whenever possible. Organic farming practices avoid or drastically reduce the use of synthetic pesticides and herbicides, which means lower toxin residues on your food.

In terms of animal products, try to source from farms that raise animals without the use of hormones and antibiotics. Also, choose wild-caught fish over farmed ones, as the latter can have higher levels of pollutants. Moreover, try to reduce your intake of processed foods, which often contain harmful additives and are packaged in materials that may leach toxins.

Lifestyle Changes to Minimize Environmental Toxin Exposure

Apart from dietary changes and product choices, you can also adopt certain lifestyle modifications to further reduce your environmental toxin exposure. One effective way is to foster indoor plants that can purify the air by absorbing harmful toxins. Plants like spider plants, snake plants, and peace lilies are known for their air-purifying abilities.

Avoid smoking and limit alcohol consumption, as these habits can introduce additional toxins into your body, burdening your detoxification system and triggering inflammation. Also, be cautious of potential environmental hazards in your workplace and ensure proper safety measures are in place to limit your exposure.

Finally, when it comes to clothing, opt for natural fibers like cotton, linen, or wool. Synthetic materials often contain chemical residues from the production process and can introduce toxins into your system through your skin.

Enhancing Detoxification Mechanisms

Even with all these efforts, some exposure to environmental toxins is inevitable. Therefore, it is equally crucial to enhance your body's natural detoxification mechanisms to effectively eliminate these toxins from your body and mitigate their inflammatory impact. Your liver, kidneys, lungs, skin, and digestive system all play crucial roles in this process.

Staying adequately hydrated, consuming a fiber-rich diet, and regular exercise can aid these processes. Hydration helps your kidneys flush toxins out of your system, while fiber binds to toxins in your digestive tract and aids in their elimination. Exercise promotes circulation and helps your skin expel toxins through sweat. Sauna use can also help enhance the elimination of toxins through perspiration.

Certain foods are known for their detoxifying properties. Cruciferous vegetables like broccoli, kale, and Brussels sprouts, for example, contain compounds that support liver detoxification. Similarly, foods rich in antioxidants, such as berries and green tea, can counteract the oxidative stress caused by toxins.

Using Natural Cleaning Products

Another major source of environmental toxins in the home is cleaning products. Many conventional cleaning products contain chemicals like phthalates, triclosan, and 2-Butoxyethanol, which are known to have detrimental health effects and can induce inflammation.

Switching to natural cleaning products can significantly reduce your exposure to these chemicals. Several brands offer eco-friendly and non-toxic cleaning products. Alternatively, you can also make your own cleaning products using ingredients like vinegar, baking soda, and essential oils, which are effective cleaners and pose minimal health risks.

Conclusion:

In essence, reducing your exposure to environmental toxins and managing inflammation requires a multifaceted approach. From the food we eat, the products we use, to the air we breathe, every aspect can contribute to or help reduce our body's toxin load. Making mindful choices in these areas can significantly help in leading a less inflammatory life. While these changes may seem small, collectively, they can make a substantial difference in your overall health and well-being. It is not just about reducing inflammation but also about fostering a healthier and more sustainable lifestyle.

8 REGULAR HEALTH CHECK-UPS

The Importance of Regular Health Checks

Regular health check-ups are a vital part of maintaining optimal health. They can help detect potential health issues before they become serious problems, enabling early intervention. They also provide an opportunity to monitor the efficacy of your anti-inflammatory lifestyle changes and make necessary adjustments. Chronic inflammation does not happen overnight, and neither does its reversal. Therefore, it is important to monitor your progress over time and stay patient and consistent with your efforts.

Understanding Inflammatory Markers

Chronic inflammation is often detected through specific blood tests that measure the levels of certain inflammation markers in your body. These markers include C-reactive protein (CRP), erythrocyte sedimentation rate (ESR), and certain cytokines. CRP is produced in response to inflammation, while ESR measures the rate at which red blood cells settle at the bottom of a test tube, which can increase with inflammation. Cytokines, on the other hand, are a group of proteins secreted by immune cells that play a crucial role in cell signaling during immune responses.

Understanding these markers and their implications is an essential first step in monitoring inflammation levels. High levels of these markers may indicate a chronic inflammatory state, while decreasing levels over time may signify the effectiveness of your anti-inflammatory interventions. Your healthcare provider can guide you through the interpretation of these results and advise you on the next steps.

Monitoring Symptoms

While blood tests can provide valuable insights into your body's inflammatory status, it is also essential to pay attention to how you feel. Symptoms like persistent fatigue, digestive issues, chronic pain, and frequent infections can all indicate chronic inflammation. Even subtle changes in these symptoms can provide important clues about the state of your inflammation. Regularly noting down these symptoms and discussing them with your healthcare provider can help paint a more comprehensive picture of your inflammation status.

The Role of Regular Screenings

In addition to monitoring inflammation levels, regular screenings for various health conditions can also play a crucial role in managing inflammation. Conditions like diabetes, heart disease, and certain types of cancer are closely associated with chronic inflammation. Regular screenings can help detect these conditions early and initiate timely treatment, thereby mitigating the effects of inflammation.

For example, regular blood pressure checks, cholesterol tests, and blood glucose tests can help monitor heart health and detect early signs of cardiovascular diseases. Similarly, regular screenings like mammograms, Pap smears, and colonoscopies can help detect certain cancers at an early stage.

Tailoring Lifestyle Changes Based on Health Checks

The results of your health checks and inflammation monitoring can provide valuable insights to tailor your lifestyle changes further. For instance, if your cholesterol levels are high, your healthcare provider may recommend a particular emphasis on dietary changes and physical activity to lower cholesterol levels. If your blood pressure is high, stress management techniques might take center stage. If certain inflammatory markers are still high, it might indicate the need for further dietary changes, more physical activity, or additional medical intervention.

Engaging Healthcare Professionals

While a lot of health management can be done independently, it is important to understand the irreplaceable role of healthcare professionals in this process. They not only interpret your health check results but also provide expert guidance on how to respond to them.

It is also beneficial to have a multidisciplinary team of healthcare professionals working with you on your journey toward an anti-inflammatory lifestyle. For instance, a nutritionist or dietitian can provide personalized dietary advice, a physiotherapist can help design an exercise regime suited to your abilities and needs, and a psychologist or counselor can assist in managing stress and mental health.

It is crucial to keep your healthcare team updated about your health status and any changes in symptoms or lifestyle. Open communication with your healthcare team can lead to better health outcomes and more effective inflammation management.

Following Up on Health Checks

A common mistake people make when it comes to health checks is failing to follow up on them. Receiving your health check results is just the first step in the process. The next crucial steps are understanding what those results mean, creating a plan of action based on them, and following through with that plan.

It would be best if you aimed to have regular follow-up appointments with your healthcare provider to discuss your health check results, understand their implications, and make any necessary adjustments to your anti-inflammatory lifestyle plan. It is important to approach these follow-ups with an open mind and a willingness to make changes if required.

Monitoring Progress Over Time

Lastly, it is crucial to understand that controlling inflammation is not a one-time task but a continuous process. Regular monitoring of inflammation levels and health checks provides the opportunity to track your progress over time.

Seeing improvements in health check results can serve as a motivating factor in maintaining lifestyle changes. Conversely, if the results are different from what is expected, do not be discouraged. It is a signal to reassess your strategies and make necessary adjustments.

Remember, overcoming chronic inflammation takes time, patience, and consistent effort. Celebrate small victories, like a slight decrease in inflammation levels or an improvement in symptoms and use any setbacks as opportunities to learn and adapt.

Closing Thoughts:

Regular health checks and monitoring inflammation levels play a pivotal role in managing and reducing chronic inflammation. They are vital in gauging the effectiveness of your anti-inflammatory lifestyle and making necessary modifications along the way. While this journey requires a proactive approach to your health and strong communication with your healthcare team, the rewards – improved health, reduced inflammation, and a better quality of life – are well worth the effort.

The regular monitoring of inflammation levels should not be viewed as a task but as an essential component of your commitment to a healthier lifestyle. Armed with the knowledge of your body's responses, you are more capable of making informed decisions, allowing you to regain control over your health.

In the next step, we will delve into the role of sleep in managing inflammation. As it turns out, getting a good night's sleep could do more than just make you feel well-rested.

9 PERSONALIZING YOUR APPROACH

The Importance of Personalization

An essential principle in effective inflammation management is that there is no 'one size fits all' approach. Each person's body is unique, their lifestyle diverse, and their personal preferences distinct. What works for one person may not necessarily work for another, and vice versa.

This uniqueness stems from differences in genetics, environmental influences, health status, and personal lifestyle choices. The journey towards an anti-inflammatory lifestyle should therefore be as unique as the individual undertaking it. Personalization is the process of tailoring the approach to suit an individual's unique needs and circumstances. It takes into consideration a range of factors, including age, gender, current health status, genetic predispositions, personal preferences, and lifestyle constraints.

Personalizing Your Diet

When it comes to diet, personalization is key. There is a broad range of dietary plans and advice out there, but not all of them will suit everyone. For some people, a plant-based diet might work well, while others may do better on a balanced diet that includes lean protein.

A personalized diet is one that takes into account your unique nutritional needs, food preferences, health status, and lifestyle. It should be nutritionally balanced, enjoyable, and sustainable in the long run.

Consider your daily routine, dietary preferences, and any pre-existing health conditions. For example, if you have high cholesterol, you might want to limit your intake of saturated fats. Or, if you are vegetarian, you will need to ensure you are getting enough protein from plant-based sources.

A professional dietician or nutritionist can help you design a personalized diet plan that suits your needs. They can guide you on portion sizes, meal timing, food preparation methods, and how to include a variety of nutrient-dense foods in your diet.

Tailoring Physical Activity

Just like diet, physical activity should also be personalized. The type, duration, intensity, and frequency of exercise that is best for you will depend on various factors. These include your current fitness level, health status, age, personal interests, and lifestyle constraints.

Remember that physical activity should be enjoyable and not feel like a chore. If you dread your workouts, it is going to be challenging to stick with them in the long run. Hence, choose activities that you enjoy and look forward to.

If you love nature, for instance, you might enjoy outdoor activities like hiking, cycling, or jogging. On the other hand, if you prefer social activities, you might want to join a dance class or a local sports club.

If you have any health conditions or physical limitations, consult with a healthcare professional before starting any new exercise routine. They can guide you on safe and effective ways to stay active.

Customizing Stress Management Techniques

Stress plays a critical role in chronic inflammation. However, what stresses one person might not stress another. Therefore, it is crucial to identify your personal stressors and find effective ways to manage them.

There are various stress management techniques available, from mindfulness and meditation to yoga and deep-breathing exercises. It is helpful to choose techniques that you find calming and enjoyable and that fit well into your lifestyle.

For instance, if you enjoy solitude and silence, you might find mindfulness meditation or quiet nature walks helpful. If you are a social person, you might prefer stress-relief activities that involve other people, such as group yoga classes or support group meetings.

In the end, personalizing your approach to stress management means being in tune with your own needs, listening to your body, and respecting your individual rhythm and pace.

Harnessing the Power of Genetic Testing

In this era of personalized medicine, genetic testing offers a fascinating tool to tailor our health strategies. By analyzing our unique genetic blueprint, these tests can provide insights into our predispositions towards certain health conditions, including those linked with inflammation, such as heart disease, arthritis, and certain types of cancer.

There are genes, for instance, that influence how we metabolize certain foods. Some people may be genetically predisposed to having an inflammatory response to certain substances like gluten or lactose. Knowing this can guide dietary choices and help avoid potential inflammatory triggers.

Similarly, genetic testing can also guide our fitness strategies. Certain genes can influence our physical traits, such as muscle composition, the propensity to gain weight, and even how we respond to different types of exercise.

However, it is important to interpret genetic testing results with caution. Genes are not our destiny. They only indicate potential risks, and these risks can be mitigated with lifestyle modifications. Professional guidance is advisable to interpret these tests and make informed health decisions.

Considering Cultural and Social Factors

Our cultural background and social environments also play a crucial role in personalizing our approach to an anti-inflammatory lifestyle. Dietary preferences, for instance, can vary significantly across different cultures.

Consider cultural adaptation when choosing your diet or other health habits. You do not have to give up your favorite ethnic dishes. Instead, look for ways to make them healthier. If a dish is typically cooked with a lot of unhealthy fats, consider using healthier cooking methods or replacing some ingredients with more nutritious options.

Our social environments also influence our lifestyle choices. If you live in an environment where fast food and sedentary behavior are the norm, it might be more challenging to adopt healthy habits. In such cases, seek social support, join health-focused community groups, or consider involving your family or friends in your health journey.

Personal Health Technology

In today's digital age, personal health technologies such as fitness trackers and health apps can help personalize and monitor our health strategies. These tools can track a variety of health parameters like daily physical activity, sleep quality, calorie intake, heart rate, and more.

Using this data can provide personalized feedback and tips. For instance, a fitness tracker might suggest that you increase your daily steps if you have been relatively inactive, or a nutrition app might point out that your diet is lacking in certain nutrients.

However, remember that these tools should be used as guides, not as definitive measures of health. They can certainly aid in self-monitoring and promoting healthy behaviors, but they are not substitutes for professional health advice.

Adopting a Patient and Flexible Mindset

Finally, remember that adopting an anti-inflammatory lifestyle is a process that takes time. It involves trial and error. What works initially might need to be tweaked as your body changes or as new research findings emerge.

Maintain a flexible mindset. If something does not work out, do not view it as a failure but rather as an opportunity to learn and adjust your approach. Celebrate small victories and progress, and do not be too hard on yourself if things do not go as planned.

Stay patient with yourself and remember that lasting changes take time. The most important thing is to remain committed to your goal of leading an anti-inflammatory lifestyle and to make consistent efforts towards achieving this goal.

10 ANTI-INFLAMMATORY LIFESTYLE

Understanding the Lifelong Commitment

Maintaining an anti-inflammatory lifestyle is indeed a lifelong commitment. It is not about quick fixes or short-term diets but a fundamental change in how you approach your health and well-being. This change involves how you eat, move, sleep, manage stress, and interact with your environment.

Change is always challenging, and it is natural to face resistance and lapses. But remember perfection is not the goal here. What matters is progress and consistency. It is about making better choices more often and gradually incorporating these changes into your lifestyle until they become second nature.

Always remember the why behind your efforts. By adopting an anti-inflammatory lifestyle, you are investing in your future health. You are lowering your risk of chronic diseases, enhancing your vitality, and improving your quality of life.

Staying Motivated: Setting Realistic Goals and Tracking Progress

Staying motivated is crucial in maintaining any lifestyle change. One effective strategy is to set realistic and specific goals. Instead of vague goals like "eat healthier," aim for specific ones like "include at least five servings of fruits and vegetables in my diet each day."

Use a health journal or a mobile app to track your progress toward these goals. This can provide a sense of achievement and keep you motivated. Remember to celebrate small victories along the way - every healthy choice you make is a step towards better health.

Overcoming Common Challenges

In your journey towards an anti-inflammatory lifestyle, you may face various challenges. These could be situational, like attending a party or dining out, where unhealthy food options are ubiquitous. Or it could be emotional challenges like stress or low mood that make you prone to unhealthy choices.

For situational challenges, plan ahead. If you're going to a party, have a small healthy snack before you go so you're not ravenous when you're faced with unhealthy choices. If dining out, consider looking up the restaurant's menu in advance and deciding on a healthy choice.

For emotional challenges, remember the stress management techniques from Step 6. Practices like mindfulness, yoga, and deep breathing can help manage emotional states and prevent stress-eating.

Also, it is important to understand that lapses are part of the process. If you have had a moment of indulgence, do not beat yourself up or let it spiral into more unhealthy choices. Acknowledge it, learn from it, and make a plan to get back on track.

Building a Supportive Environment

Our environment greatly influences our behaviors. Make your environment supportive of your anti-inflammatory lifestyle. This could mean stocking up your kitchen with anti-inflammatory foods, setting up a corner in your home for exercise, or even digital reminders to take a break from work and relax.

Another powerful strategy is to involve others in your journey. Having a friend with similar health goals can provide mutual encouragement and make the process more enjoyable. You could also involve your family in your health goals - this not only gives you support but also promotes the health of your loved ones.

Lifelong Learning

Stay informed about the latest research in inflammation and health. Science is constantly evolving, and new findings may offer more insights to fine-tune your anti-inflammatory strategies. However, always be critical of the information you read, especially online. Rely on trusted sources, and when in doubt, seek professional advice.

Remaining Resilient and Flexible

It is vital to remember that your anti-inflammatory lifestyle should be resilient and flexible. Resilience does not imply a stiff, unyielding commitment to a specific diet or routine. It is the ability to bounce back from setbacks, to learn from them, and to continue to move forward. Flexibility allows you to adjust your strategies according to the changing circumstances, needs, and stages of your life. Remember, an anti-inflammatory lifestyle is not a strict set of rules but a guiding principle that you can adapt to serve your unique lifestyle and health needs.

Recognizing Individuality in Health

Everyone's health experience is unique, and comparison can be a significant demotivator. It is essential to recognize and respect your individual path and progress. Your body's response to inflammation and its interaction with various anti-inflammatory strategies will be unique to you.

Remember, there is no universal timeline for health improvements. It could take weeks or even months to see noticeable changes. Patience and persistence are vital. Focus on how you feel — improved energy levels, better mood, or better sleep — these are all signs of your body healing from the inside.

Continuing Education and Consultation

Never underestimate the power of knowledge and consultation. Continue educating yourself about new developments in the field of inflammation, nutrition, and lifestyle modifications. Always refer to scientifically backed sources or consult with healthcare professionals.

Consider regular consultations with a healthcare provider who understands your journey towards an anti-inflammatory lifestyle. Regular check-ups and health screenings can help monitor your progress and adjust your strategies as needed. They can also provide motivation and reassurance and address any concerns or obstacles you might encounter.

Creating an Anti-Inflammatory Community

Building a community around your new lifestyle can be incredibly helpful in maintaining the lifestyle changes. This could be friends, family, or even online communities of people who are also striving for an anti-inflammatory lifestyle. Sharing experiences, tips, recipes, or just mutual encouragement can make the experience less daunting and more enjoyable.

A Lifelong Anti-Inflammatory Lifestyle

Achieving an anti-inflammatory lifestyle is essentially a commitment to your future self. It is a commitment to invest in your health today to enjoy the benefits of vitality and wellness in the years to come.

Remember, this journey is not just about preventing or managing diseases but about improving your quality of life.

It is about enabling you to do more of what you love and less of what you do not.

With every step you take, you are adding life to your years and years to your life. You are embracing a lifestyle that supports your body's natural ability to heal and thrive. By the end of these ten steps, you have not only gained a profound understanding of inflammation and its impact on your health, but you have also equipped yourself with practical strategies and techniques to lead a healthier, inflammation-free life.

Though the ten steps have now been explained, your journey is not over. Indeed, it is just the beginning. Continue to learn, adapt, and grow. The path may take some work, and there may be challenges along the way. But with every step you take, you are moving closer to your goal of living a healthier, more vibrant life.

SUMMARY

Anti-Inflammatory Living

Understanding and mitigating inflammation is multifaceted, spanning various aspects of our lives, from diet to physical activity, stress management, and environmental interactions. This wrap-up presents a concise yet comprehensive summary of the ten steps in our journey to an anti-inflammatory lifestyle, combining knowledge from expert sources with practical strategies and techniques.

Step 1: Understanding Inflammation

Understanding inflammation is the cornerstone to unraveling an anti-inflammatory lifestyle. Inflammation is the body's natural response to injury or illness, functioning as a biological warning system to facilitate healing. However, when this response becomes chronic, it can result in deleterious health effects and contribute to various ailments such as heart disease, diabetes, cancer, and neurodegenerative diseases. Recognizing the role of inflammation in these conditions arms us with the knowledge needed to combat it effectively.

Step 2: Recognizing Inflammatory Triggers

To control inflammation, it is essential to identify its triggers, which can span various facets of our lives. These triggers can range from our food choices, lack of physical activity, and unmanaged stress to environmental exposures such as toxins and pollutants. Recognizing these triggers is pivotal to minimizing their impact and managing inflammation.

Step 3: Adopting an Anti-Inflammatory Diet

Diet plays a central role in managing inflammation. Certain foods, like processed foods, sugars, and certain fats, can exacerbate inflammation, while others, such as fruits, vegetables, whole grains, lean proteins, and healthy fats, can reduce it. This step is about understanding and embracing an anti-inflammatory diet that nourishes our bodies and supports our health.

Step 4: Planning and Preparing Anti-Inflammatory Meals

Armed with knowledge about the anti-inflammatory diet, the next step involves practical application: planning and preparing meals that are healthy, delicious, and nourishing. This process encourages enjoyment and creativity, making the lifestyle change not only beneficial but also sustainable and enjoyable.

Step 5: Integrating Physical Activity

Physical activity, a critical element of an anti-inflammatory lifestyle, benefits our bodies in multiple ways, including reducing inflammation. This step explores how to incorporate various forms of exercise into our routines, ensuring they are manageable, enjoyable, and beneficial in promoting an anti-inflammatory state.

Step 6: Managing Stress

Chronic stress can exacerbate inflammation, making stress management a vital part of the anti-inflammatory lifestyle. This step delves into various stress-management techniques, from mindfulness and meditation to yoga and relaxation exercises, and their efficacy in controlling inflammation.

Step 7: Reducing Exposure to Environmental Inflammation Triggers

Our environment can also contribute to inflammation, especially when we are exposed to pollutants and toxins. This step guides us to minimize our exposure, helping us lead healthier, cleaner lives and further reduce inflammation.

Step 8: Regular Health Check-ups and Monitoring Inflammation Levels

Regular health check-ups can help detect early signs of chronic inflammation and monitor the effectiveness of our anti-inflammatory lifestyle. This step provides guidance on what to look for and how to interpret health metrics related to inflammation.

Step 9: Personalizing Your Approach

Each individual is unique, necessitating a personalized approach to an anti-inflammatory lifestyle. This step encourages tailoring diet, physical activity, and stress management techniques to individual needs, preferences, and lifestyles, promoting a more effective and enjoyable experience towards anti-inflammatory living.

Step 10: Maintaining the Anti-Inflammatory Lifestyle

The final step addresses sustainability. Adopting an anti-inflammatory lifestyle is a lifelong commitment, not a short-term undertaking. This step offers strategies to stay motivated and tips to overcome common challenges, ensuring long-term adherence and success.

By following these ten steps, we gain not only a comprehensive understanding of inflammation and its impacts on health but also a practical toolkit to lead a healthier, inflammation-free life. The ultimate aim of this journey is to add not just years to our lives but life to our years, enabling us to enjoy good health and vitality for as long as possible. This approach represents a holistic approach to health and wellness, underscoring the interconnectedness of various lifestyle factors and their cumulative impact on our well-being.

10 Steps for Reducing Inflammation

Made in the USA
Las Vegas, NV
04 February 2024

85240983R00046